# Heroin

# Table of Contents

**Heroin**

Letter From the Director

What is heroin and how is it used?

What is the scope of heroin use in the United States?

What effects does heroin have on the body?

What are the immediate (short-term) effects of heroin use?

What are the long-term effects of heroin use?

How is heroin linked to prescription drug abuse?

What are the medical complications of chronic heroin use?

Why does heroin use create special risk for contracting HIV/AIDS and hepatitis B and C?

How does heroin use affect pregnant women?

What can be done for a heroin overdose?

What are the treatments for heroin addiction?

Where can I get further information about heroin?

Glossary

References

# Letter From the Director

Heroin is a highly addictive opioid drug, and its use has repercussions that extend far beyond the individual user. The medical and social consequences of drug use—such as hepatitis, HIV/AIDS, fetal effects, crime, violence, and disruptions in family, workplace, and educational environments—have a devastating impact on society and cost billions of dollars each year.

Although heroin use in the general population is rather low, the numbers of people starting to use heroin have been steadily rising since 2007.[1] This may be due in part to a shift from abuse of prescription pain relievers to heroin as a readily available, cheaper alternative[2-5] and the misperception that highly pure heroin is safer than less pure forms because it does not need to be injected.

Like many other chronic diseases, addiction can be treated. Medications are available to treat heroin addiction while reducing drug cravings and withdrawal symptoms, improving the odds of achieving abstinence. There are now a variety of medications that can be tailored to a person's recovery needs while taking into account co-occurring health conditions. Medication combined with behavioral therapy is particularly effective, offering hope to individuals who suffer from addiction and for those around them.

The National Institute on Drug Abuse (NIDA) has developed this publication to provide an overview of heroin use and its consequences as well as treatment options available for those struggling with heroin addiction. We hope this compilation of scientific information on heroin will help to inform readers about the harmful effects of heroin as well as assist in prevention and treatment efforts.

**Nora D. Volkow, M.D.**
Director
National Institute on Drug Abuse

# What is heroin and how is it used?

Heroin is an illegal, highly addictive drug processed from morphine, a naturally occurring substance extracted from the seed pod of certain varieties of poppy plants. It is typically sold as a white or brownish powder that is "cut" with sugars, starch, powdered milk, or quinine. Pure heroin is a white powder with a bitter taste that predominantly originates in South America and, to a lesser extent, from Southeast Asia, and dominates U.S. markets east of the Mississippi River.[3] Highly pure heroin can be snorted or smoked and may be more appealing to new users because it eliminates the stigma associated with injection drug use. "Black tar" heroin is sticky like roofing tar or hard like coal and is predominantly produced in Mexico and sold in U.S. areas west of the Mississippi River.[3] The dark color associated with black tar heroin results from crude processing methods that leave behind impurities. Impure heroin is usually dissolved, diluted, and injected into veins, muscles, or under the skin.

# What is the scope of heroin use in the United States?

According to the National Survey on Drug Use and Health (NSDUH), in 2016 about 948,000 Americans reported using heroin in the past year,[1] a number that has been on the rise since 2007. This trend appears to be driven largely by young adults aged 18–25 among whom there have been the greatest increases. The number of people using heroin for the first time is unacceptably high, with 170,000 people starting heroin use in 2016, nearly double the number of people in 2006 (90,000). In contrast, heroin use has been declining among teens aged 12–17. Past-year heroin use among the Nation's 8th-, 10th-, and 12th-graders is at its lowest levels in the history of the Monitoring the Future survey, at less than 1 percent of those surveyed in all 3 grades from 2005 to 2017.[6]

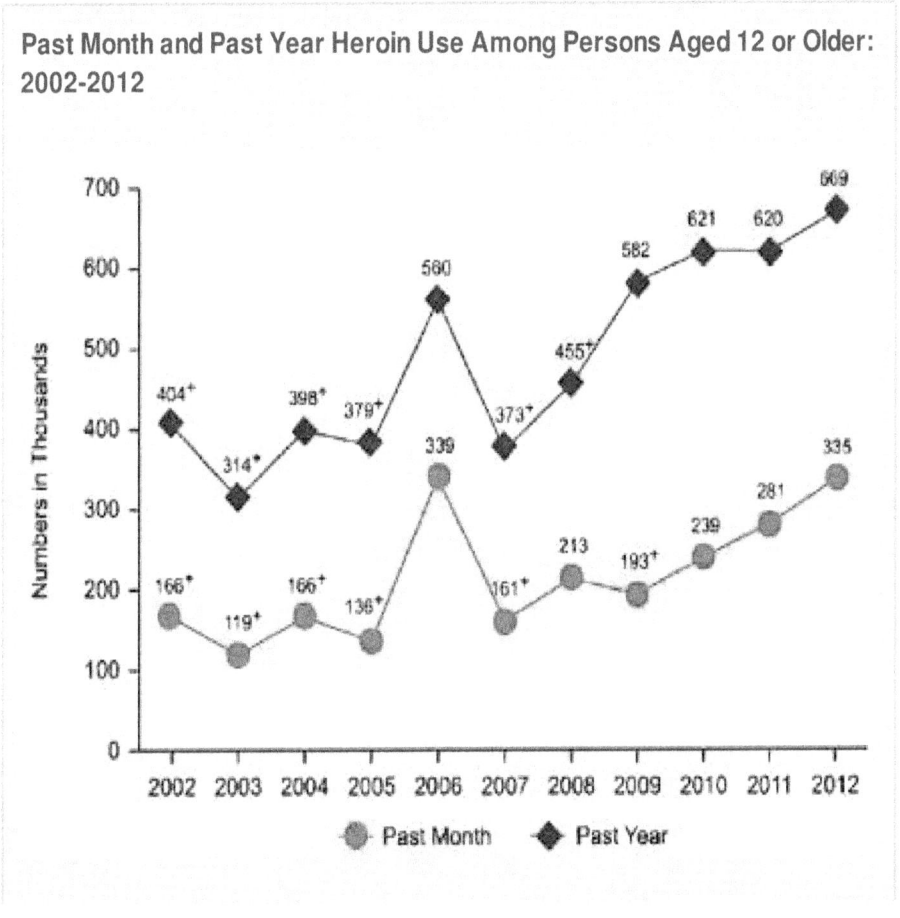

Past Month and Past Year Heroin Use Among Persons Aged 12 or Older: 2002-2012

Source: National Survey on Drug Use and Health: Summary of National Findings, 2012.

It is no surprise that with heroin use on the rise, more people are experiencing negative health effects that occur from repeated use. The number of people meeting Diagnostic and Statistical Manual of Mental Disorders, 4th edition (DSM-IV) criteria for dependence or abuse of heroin increased dramatically from 214,000 in 2002 to 626,000 in 2016.[1] The recently released DSM-V no longer separates substance abuse from dependence, but instead provides criteria for opioid use disorders that range from mild to severe, depending on the number of symptoms a person has.[7] Data on the scope and severity of opioid use disorders in the United States are not yet available for these new criteria.

The impact of heroin use is felt all across the United States, with heroin being identified as the most or one of the most important drug abuse issues affecting several local regions from coast to coast. The rising harm associated with heroin use at the community level was presented in a report produced by the NIDA Community Epidemiology Work Group (CEWG). The CEWG is comprised of researchers from major metropolitan areas in the United States and selected foreign countries and provides community-level surveillance of drug abuse and its consequences to identify emerging trends.[3]

Heroin use no longer predominates solely in urban areas. Several suburban and rural communities near Chicago and St. Louis report increasing amounts of heroin seized by officials as well as increasing numbers of overdose deaths due to heroin use. Heroin use is also on the rise in many urban areas among young adults aged 18-25.[8] Individuals in this age group seeking treatment for heroin abuse increased from 11 percent of total admissions in 2008 to 26 percent in the first half of 2012.

# What effects does heroin have on the body?

> The greatest increase in heroin use is seen in young adults aged 18-25.

Heroin binds to and activates specific receptors in the brain called mu-opioid receptors (MORs). Our bodies contain naturally occurring chemicals called neurotransmitters that bind to these receptors throughout the brain and body to regulate pain, hormone release, and feelings of well-being.[9] When MORs are activated in the reward center of the brain, they stimulate the release of the neurotransmitter dopamine, causing a sensation of pleasure.[10] The consequences of activating opioid receptors with externally administered opioids such as heroin (versus naturally occurring chemicals within our bodies) depend on a variety of factors: how much is used, where in the brain or body it binds, how strongly it binds and for how long, how quickly it gets there, and what happens afterward.

# What are the immediate (short-term) effects of heroin use?

Once heroin enters the brain, it is converted to morphine and binds rapidly to opioid receptors.[11] Abusers typically report feeling a surge of pleasurable sensation—a "rush." The intensity of the rush is a function of how much drug is taken and how rapidly the drug enters the brain and binds to the opioid receptors. With heroin, the rush is usually accompanied by a warm flushing of the skin, dry mouth, and a heavy feeling in the extremities, which may be accompanied by nausea, vomiting, and severe itching. After the initial effects, users usually will be drowsy for several hours; mental function is clouded; heart function slows; and breathing is also severely slowed, sometimes enough to be life-threatening. Slowed breathing can also lead to coma and permanent brain damage.[12]

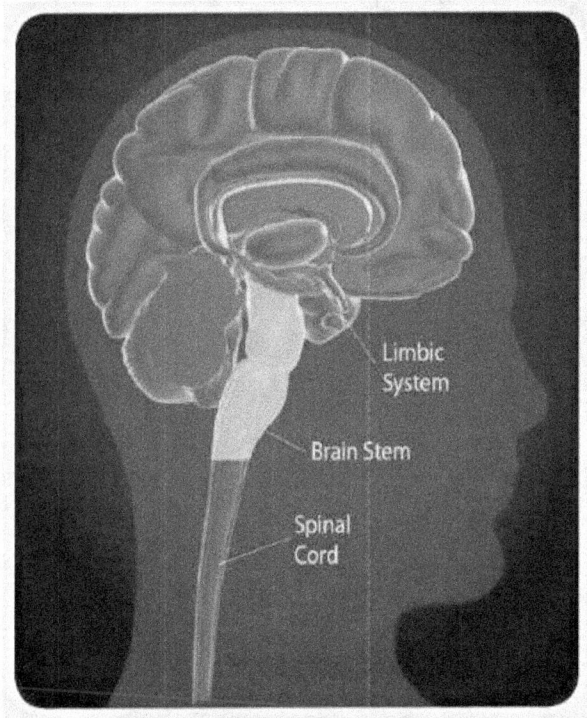

**Opioids Act on Many Places in the Brain and Nervous System**

- Opioids can depress breathing by changing neurochemical activity in the brain stem, where automatic body functions such as breathing and heart rate are controlled.

- Opioids can increase feelings of pleasure by altering activity in the limbic system, which controls emotions.

- Opioids can block pain messages transmitted through the spinal cord from the body.

# What are the long-term effects of heroin use?

Repeated heroin use changes the physical structure[13] and physiology of the brain, creating long-term imbalances in neuronal and hormonal systems that are not easily reversed.[14,15] Studies have shown some deterioration of the brain's white matter due to heroin use, which may affect decision-making abilities, the ability to regulate behavior, and responses to stressful situations.[16-18] Heroin also produces profound degrees of tolerance and physical dependence. Tolerance occurs when more and more of the drug is required to achieve the same effects. With physical dependence, the body adapts to the presence of the drug and withdrawal symptoms occur if use is reduced abruptly. Withdrawal may occur within a few hours after the last time the drug is taken. Symptoms of withdrawal include restlessness, muscle and bone pain, insomnia, diarrhea, vomiting, cold flashes with goose bumps ("cold turkey"), and leg movements. Major withdrawal symptoms peak between 24–48 hours after the last dose of heroin and subside after about a week. However, some people have shown persistent withdrawal signs for many months. Finally, repeated heroin use often results in addiction—a chronic relapsing disease that goes beyond physical dependence and is characterized by uncontrollable drug-seeking no matter the consequences.[19] Heroin is extremely addictive no matter how it is administered, although routes of administration that allow it to reach the brain the fastest (i.e., injection and smoking) increase the risk of addiction. Once a person becomes addicted to heroin, seeking and using the drug becomes their primary purpose in life.

# How is heroin linked to prescription drug abuse?

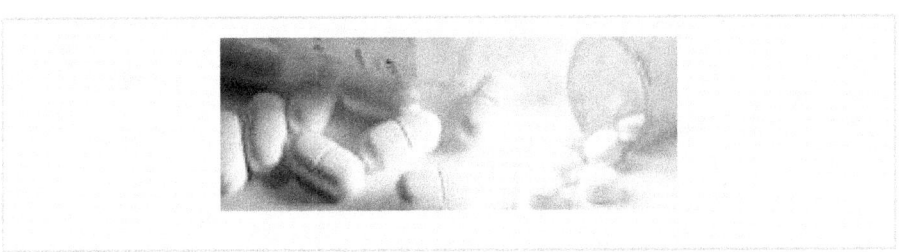

Harmful health consequences resulting from the abuse of opioid medications that are prescribed for the treatment of pain, such as Oxycontin®, Vicodin®, and Demerol®, have dramatically increased in recent years. For example, unintentional poisoning deaths from prescription opioids quadrupled from 1999 to 2010 and now outnumber those from heroin and cocaine combined.[20] People often assume prescription pain relievers are safer than illicit drugs because they are medically prescribed; however, when these drugs are taken for reasons or in ways or amounts not intended by a doctor, or taken by someone other than the person for whom they are prescribed, they can result in severe adverse health effects including addiction, overdose, and death, especially when combined with other drugs or alcohol. Research now suggests that abuse of these medications may actually open the door to heroin use. Nearly half of young people who inject heroin surveyed in three recent studies reported abusing prescription opioids before starting to use heroin. Some individuals reported switching to heroin because it is cheaper and easier to obtain than prescription opioids.[2-4]

# What are the medical complications of chronic heroin use?

**Short- and Long-Term Effects of Heroin Use**

**Short-Term Effects**

- "Rush"
- Depressed respiration
- Clouded mental functioning
- Nausea and vomiting
- Suppression of pain
- Spontaneous abortion

**Long-Term Effects**

- Addiction
- Infectious disease (e.g., HIV, hepatitis B and C)
- Collapsed veins
- Bacterial infections
- Abscesses
- Infection of heart lining and valves
- Arthritis and other rheumatologic problems
- Liver and kidney disease

No matter how they ingest the drug, chronic heroin users experience a variety of medical complications including insomnia and constipation. Lung complications (including various types of pneumonia and tuberculosis) may result from the poor health of the user as well as from heroin's effect of depressing respiration. Many experience mental disorders such as depression and antisocial personality disorder. Men often experience sexual dysfunction and women's menstrual cycles often become irregular. There are also specific consequences associated with different routes of administration. For example, people who repeatedly snort heroin can damage the mucosal tissues in their noses as well as perforate the nasal septum (the tissue that separates the nasal passages).

Medical consequences of chronic injection use include scarred and/or collapsed veins, bacterial infections of the blood vessels and heart valves, abscesses (boils), and other soft-tissue infections. Many of the additives in street heroin may include substances that do not readily dissolve and result in clogging the blood vessels that lead to the lungs, liver, kidneys, or brain. This can cause infection or even death of small patches of cells in vital organs. Immune reactions to these or other contaminants can cause arthritis or other rheumatologic problems.

Sharing of injection equipment or fluids can lead to some of the most severe consequences of heroin abuse—infections with hepatitis B and C, HIV, and a host of other blood-borne viruses, which drug abusers can then pass on to their sexual partners and children.

# Why does heroin use create special risk for contracting HIV/AIDS and hepatitis B and C?

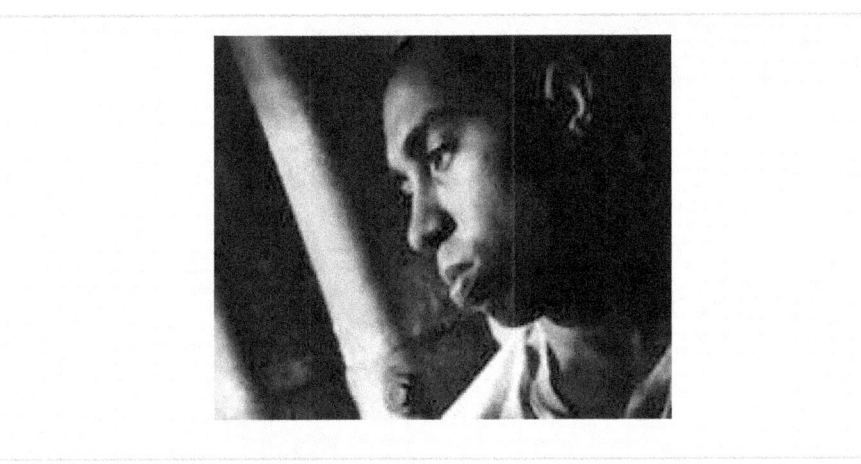

Heroin use increases the risk of being exposed to HIV, viral hepatitis, and other infectious agents through contact with infected blood or body fluids (e.g., semen, saliva) that results from the sharing of syringes and injection paraphernalia that have been used by infected individuals or through unprotected sexual contact with an infected person. Snorting or smoking does not eliminate the risk of infectious disease like hepatitis and HIV/AIDS because people under the influence of drugs still engage in risky sexual and other behaviors that can expose them to these diseases.

Injection drug users (IDUs) are the highest-risk group for acquiring hepatitis C (HCV) infection and continue to drive the escalating HCV epidemic: Each IDU infected with HCV is likely to infect 20 other people.[21] Of the 17,000 new HCV infections occurring in the United States in 2010, over half (53 percent) were among IDUs.[22] Hepatitis B (HBV) infection in IDUs was reported to be as high as 20 percent in the United States in 2010,[23] which is particularly disheartening since an effective vaccine that protects against HBV infection is available. There is currently no vaccine available to protect against HCV infection.

Drug use, viral hepatitis and other infectious diseases, mental illnesses, social dysfunctions, and stigma are often co-occuring conditions that affect one another, creating more complex health challenges that require comprehensive treatment plans tailored to meet all of a patient's needs. For example, NIDA-funded research has found that drug abuse treatment along with HIV prevention and community-based outreach programs can help people who use drugs change the behaviors that put them at risk for contracting HIV and other infectious diseases. They can reduce drug use and drug-related risk behaviors such as needle sharing and unsafe sexual practices and, in turn, reduce the risk of exposure to HIV/AIDS and other infectious diseases. Only through coordinated utilization of effective antiviral therapies coupled with treatment for drug abuse and mental illness can the health of those suffering from these conditions be restored.

# How does heroin use affect pregnant women?

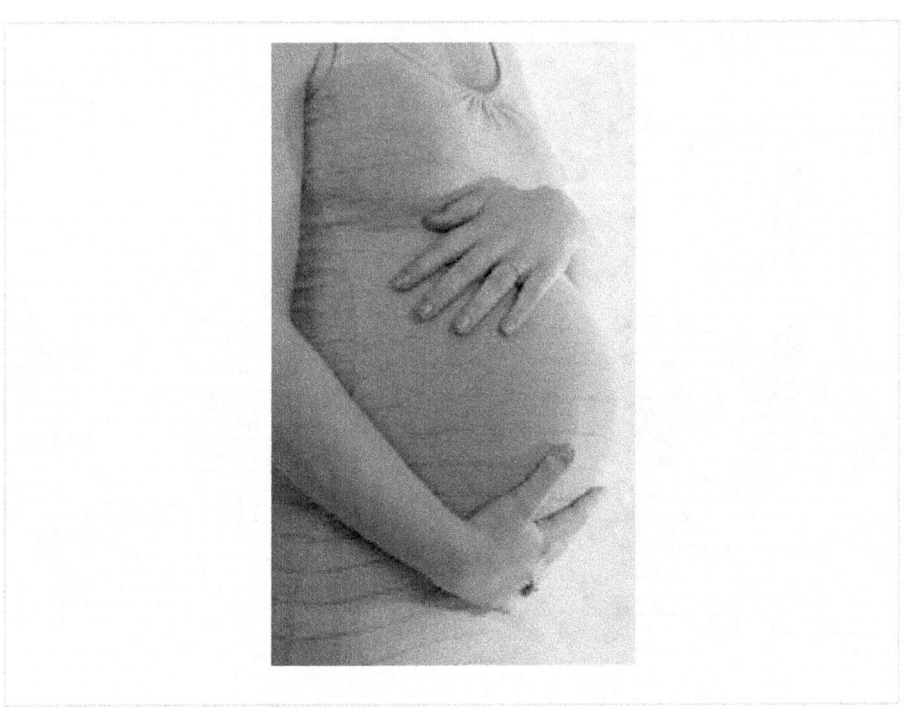

Heroin use during pregnancy can result in neonatal abstinence syndrome (NAS). NAS occurs when heroin passes through the placenta to the fetus during pregnancy, causing the baby to become dependent along with the mother. Symptoms include excessive crying, fever, irritability, seizures, slow weight gain, tremors, diarrhea, vomiting, and possibly death. NAS requires hospitalization and treatment with medication (often morphine) to relieve symptoms; the medication is gradually tapered off until the baby adjusts to being opioid-free. Methadone maintenance combined with prenatal care and a comprehensive drug treatment program can improve many of the outcomes associated with untreated heroin use for both the infant and mother, although infants exposed to methadone during pregnancy typically require treatment for NAS as well.

A recent NIDA-supported clinical trial demonstrated that buprenorphine treatment of opioid-dependent mothers is safe for both the unborn child and the mother. Once born, these infants require less morphine and shorter hospital stays as compared to infants born of mothers on methadone maintenance treatment.[24]

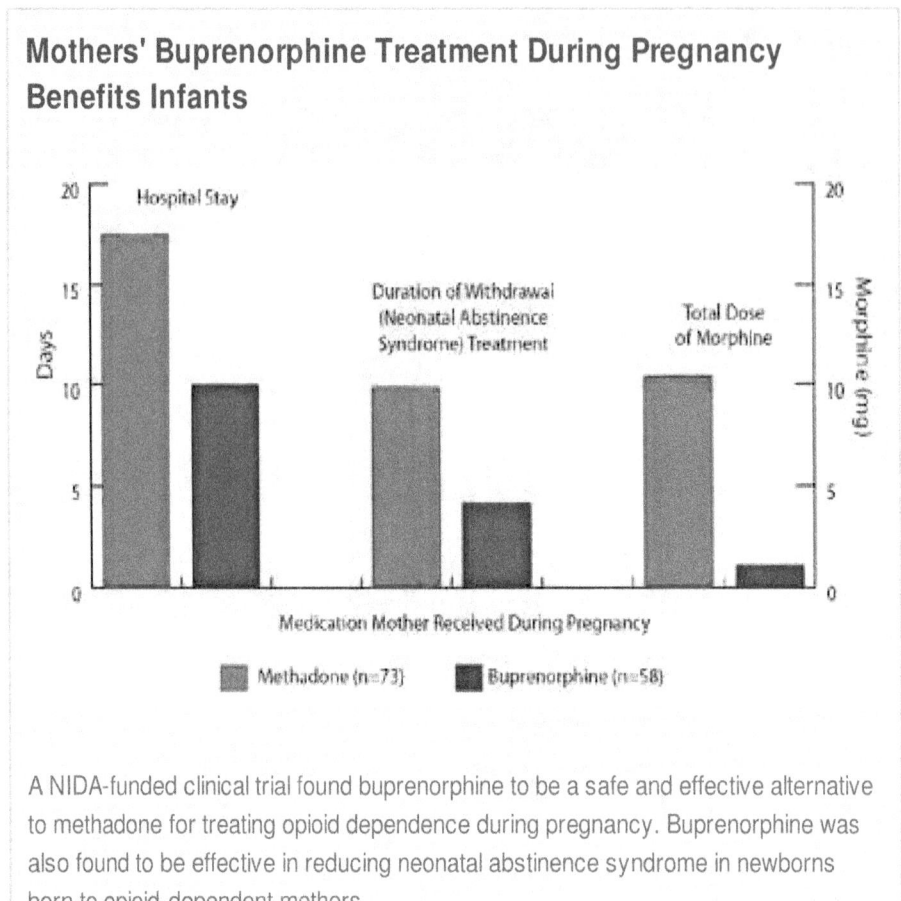

A NIDA-funded clinical trial found buprenorphine to be a safe and effective alternative to methadone for treating opioid dependence during pregnancy. Buprenorphine was also found to be effective in reducing neonatal abstinence syndrome in newborns born to opioid-dependent mothers.

Research indicates that buprenorphine combined with naloxone (compared to a morphine taper) is equally safe for treating babies born with NAS, further reducing side effects experienced by infants born to opioid-dependent mothers.[25,26] There is some evidence that buprenorphine is superior to morphine in treating infants with NAS. A NIDA-funded study published in June 2017 found that treating NAS babies with sublingual buprenorphine resulted in a shorter duration of treatment than oral morphine, and also resulted in a shorter length of hospital stay, with similar rates of adverse events.

# What can be done for a heroin overdose?

Overdose is a dangerous and deadly consequence of heroin use. A large dose of heroin depresses heart rate and breathing to such an extent that a user cannot survive without medical help. Naloxone (e.g., Narcan®) is an opioid receptor antagonist medication that can eliminate all signs of opioid intoxication to reverse an opioid overdose. It works by rapidly binding to opioid receptors, preventing heroin from activating them.[27] Because of the huge increase in overdose deaths from prescription opioid abuse, there has been greater demand for opioid overdose prevention services. Naloxone that can be used by nonmedical personnel has been shown to be cost-effective and save lives.[28] In April 2014, the U.S. Food and Drug Administration (FDA) approved a naloxone hand-held auto-injector called Evzio, which rapidly delivers a single dose of naloxone into the muscle or under the skin, buying time until medical assistance can arrive. Since Evzio can be used by family members or caregivers, it greatly expands access to naloxone.[29] NIDA and the FDA are working with drug manufacturers to support the development of nasal spray formulations of this live-saving medication.

In addition, the Substance Abuse and Mental Health Services Administration (SAMHSA) released an Opioid Overdose Prevention Toolkit in August 2013 that provides helpful information necessary to develop policies and practices to prevent opioid-related overdoses and deaths. The kit provides material tailored for first responders, treatment providers, and individuals recovering from an opioid overdose.

# What are the treatments for heroin addiction?

A variety of effective treatments are available for heroin addiction, including both behavioral and pharmacological (medications). Both approaches help to restore a degree of normalcy to brain function and behavior, resulting in increased employment rates and lower risk of HIV and other diseases and criminal behavior. Although behavioral and pharmacologic treatments can be extremely useful when utilized alone, research shows that for some people, integrating both types of treatments is the most effective approach.

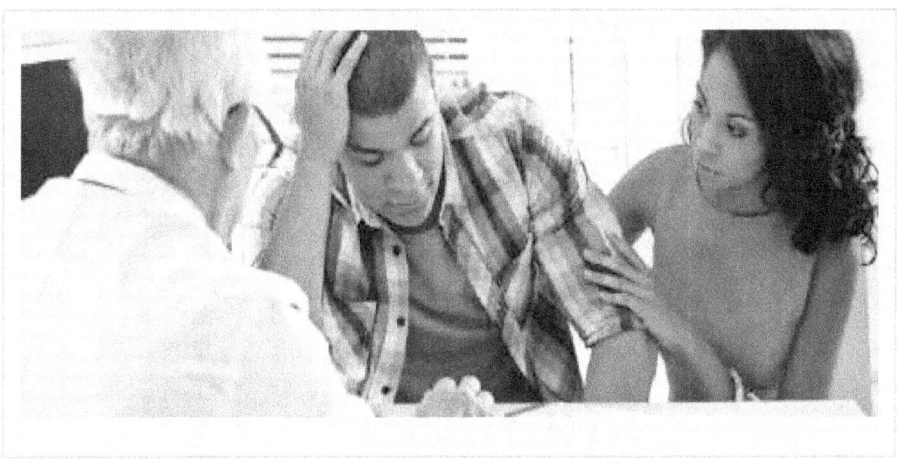

## Pharmacological Treatment (Medications)

Scientific research has established that pharmacological treatment of opioid addiction increases retention in treatment programs and decreases drug use, infectious disease transmission, and criminal activity.

When people addicted to opioids first quit, they undergo withdrawal symptoms (pain, diarrhea, nausea, and vomiting), which may be severe. Medications can be helpful in this detoxification stage to ease craving and other physical symptoms, which often prompt a person to relapse. While not a treatment for addiction itself, detoxification is a useful first step when it is followed by some form of evidence-based treatment.

Medications developed to treat opioid addiction work through the same opioid receptors as the addictive drug, but are safer and less likely to produce the harmful behaviors that characterize addiction. Three types of medications include: (1) agonists, which activate opioid receptors; (2) partial agonists, which also activate opioid receptors but produce a smaller response; and (3) antagonists, which block the receptor and interfere with the rewarding effects of opioids. A particular medication is used based on a patient's specific medical needs and other factors. Effective medications include:

- Methadone (Dolophine® or Methadose®) is a slow-acting opioid agonist. Methadone is taken orally so that it reaches the brain slowly, dampening the "high" that occurs with other routes of administration while preventing withdrawal symptoms. Methadone has been used since the 1960s to treat heroin addiction and is still an excellent treatment option, particularly for patients who do not respond well to other medications. Methadone is only available through approved outpatient treatment programs, where it is dispensed to patients on a daily basis.

- Buprenorphine (Subutex®) is a partial opioid agonist. Buprenorphine relieves drug cravings without producing the "high" or dangerous side effects of other opioids. Suboxone® is a novel formulation of buprenorphine that is taken orally or sublingually and contains naloxone (an opioid antagonist) to prevent attempts to get high by injecting the medication. If an addicted patient were to inject Suboxone, the naloxone would induce withdrawal symptoms, which are averted when taken orally as prescribed. FDA approved buprenorphine in 2002, making it the first medication eligible to be prescribed by certified physicians through the Drug Addiction Treatment Act. This approval eliminates the need to visit specialized treatment clinics, thereby expanding access to treatment for many who need it. In February 2013, FDA approved two generic forms of Suboxone, making this treatment option more affordable. In May 2016, FDA approved a 6-month subdermal buprenorphine implant and in November 2017, a once-monthly buprenorphine injection.

- Naltrexone (Depade® or Revia®) is an opioid antagonist. Naltrexone blocks the action of opioids, is not addictive or sedating, and does not result in physical dependence; however, patients often have trouble complying with the treatment, and this has limited its effectiveness. An injectable long-acting formulation of naltrexone (Vivitrol®) recently received FDA approval for treating opioid addiction. Administered once a month, Vivitrol® may improve compliance by eliminating the need for daily dosing.

A NIDA study shows that once treatment is initiated, a buprenorphine/naloxone combination and an extended release naltrexone formulation are similarly effective in treating opioid use disorder. Because naltrexone requires full detoxification, initiating treatment among active opioid users was more difficult with this medication. However, once detoxification was complete, the naltrexone formulation had a similar effectiveness as the buprenorphine/naloxone combination.

## Behavioral Therapies

The many effective behavioral treatments available for heroin addiction can be delivered in outpatient and residential settings. Approaches such as contingency management and cognitive-behavioral therapy have been shown to effectively treat heroin addiction, especially when applied in concert with medications. Contingency management uses a voucher-based system in which patients earn "points" based on negative drug tests, which they can exchange for items that encourage healthy living. Cognitive-behavioral therapy is designed to help modify the patient's expectations and behaviors related to drug use and to increase skills in coping with various life stressors. An important task is to match the best treatment approach to meet the particular needs of the patient.

# Where can I get further information about heroin?

To learn more about heroin and other drugs of abuse, visit the NIDA Web site at www.drugabuse.gov or contact the *DrugPubs* Research Dissemination Center at 877-NIDA-NIH (877-643-2644; TTY/TDD: 240-645-0228).

### What's on the NIDA Web Site

- Information on drugs of abuse and related health consequences
- NIDA publications, news, and events
- Resources for health care professionals
- Funding information (including program announcements and deadlines)
- International activities
- Links to related Web sites (access to Web sites of many other organizations in the field)

### NIDA Web Sites

- www.drugabuse.gov
- www.teens.drugabuse.gov
- www.drugabuse.gov/drugs-abuse/heroin
- www.easyread.drugabuse.gov
- www.drugabuse.gov/publications/principles-adolescent-substance-use-disorder-treatment-research-based-guide

### Other Resources

Information on heroin and addiction is also available through these other Web sites:

- Medication-Assisted Treatment for Opioid Addiction: www.drugabuse.gov/publications/topics-in-brief/medication-assisted-treatment-opioid-addiction

- Prescription Drugs: www.drugabuse.gov/drugs-abuse/prescription-drugs

- Medication-Assisted Treatment for Opioid Addiction: www.samhsa.gov/samhsaNewsLetter/Volume_17_Number_5/TreatingOpioidAddiction

---

This publication is available for your use and may be reproduced **in its entirety** without permission from the NIDA. Citation of the source is appreciated, using the following language: Source: National Institute on Drug Abuse; National Institutes of Health; U.S. Department of Health and Human Services.

# Glossary

**Addiction:** A chronic, relapsing disease, characterized by compulsive drug seeking and use accompanied by neurochemical and molecular changes in the brain.

**Agonist:** A chemical compound that mimics the action of a natural neurotransmitter and binds to the same receptor on nerve cells to produce a biological response.

**Antagonist:** A drug that binds to the same nerve cell receptor as the natural neurotransmitter but does not activate the receptor, instead blocking the effects of another drug.

**Buprenorphine:** A partial opioid agonist for the treatment of opioid addiction that relieves drug cravings without producing the "high" or dangerous side effects of other opioids.

**Craving:** A powerful, often uncontrollable desire for drugs.

**Detoxification:** A process of allowing the body to rid itself of a drug while managing the symptoms of withdrawal; often the first step in a drug treatment program.

**Methadone:** A long-acting opioid agonist medication shown to be effective in treating heroin addiction.

**Naloxone:** An opioid receptor antagonist that rapidly binds to opioid receptors, blocking heroin from activating them. An appropriate dose of naloxone acts in less than 2 minutes and completely eliminates all signs of opioid intoxication to reverse an opioid overdose.

**Naltrexone:** An opioid antagonist medication that can only be used after a patient has completed detoxification. Naltrexone is not addictive or sedating and does not result in physical dependence; however, poor patient compliance has limited its effectiveness. A new, long-acting form of naltrexone called Vivitrol® is now available that is injected once per month, eliminating the need for daily dosing, improving patient compliance.

**Neonatal abstinence syndrome (NAS):** NAS occurs when heroin from the mother passes through the placenta into the baby's bloodstream during pregnancy, allowing the baby to become addicted along with the mother. NAS requires hospitalization and treatment with medication (often a morphine taper) to relieve symptoms until the baby adjusts to becoming opioid-free.

**Opioid:** A natural or synthetic psychoactive chemical that binds to opioid receptors in the brain and body. Natural opioids include morphine and heroin (derived from the opium poppy) as well as opioids produced by the human body (e.g., endorphins); semi-synthetic or synthetic opioids include analgesics such as oxycodone, hydrocodone, and fentanyl.

**Opioid use disorder:** A problematic pattern of opioid drug use, leading to clinically significant impairment or distress that includes cognitive, behavioral, and physiological symptoms as defined by the new Diagnostic and Statistical Manual of Mental Disorders, 5th edition (DSM-V) criteria. Diagnosis of an opioid use disorder can be mild, moderate, or severe depending on the number of symptoms a person experiences. Tolerance or withdrawal symptoms that occur during medically supervised treatment are specifically excluded from an opioid use disorder diagnosis.

**Partial agonist:** A substance that binds to and activates the same nerve cell receptor as a natural neurotransmitter but produces a diminished biological response.

**Physical dependence:** An adaptive physiological state that occurs with regular drug use and results in a withdrawal syndrome when drug use is stopped; usually occurs with tolerance.

**Rush:** A surge of euphoric pleasure that rapidly follows administration of a drug.

**Tolerance:** A condition in which higher doses of a drug are required to produce the same effect as during initial use; often leads to physical dependence.

**Withdrawal:** A variety of symptoms that occur after use of an addictive drug is reduced or stopped.

# References

1. Substance Abuse Center for Behavioral Health Statistics and Quality. Results from the 2016 National Survey on Drug Use and Health: Detailed Tables. SAMHSA. https://www.samhsa.gov/data/sites/default/files/NSDUH-DetTabs-2016/NSDUH-DetTabs-2016.htm. Published September 7, 2017. Accessed March 7, 2018.

2. Cicero, T.J.; Ellis, M.S.; and Surratt, H.L. Effect of abuse-deterrent formulation of OxyContin. *N Engl J Med* 367(2):187–189, 2012.

3. National Institute on Drug Abuse. Epidemiologic Trends in Drug Abuse, in *Proceedings of the Community Epidemiology Work Group*, January 2012. Bethesda, MD: National Institute on Drug Abuse, 66.

4. Pollini, R.A.; Banta-Green, C.J.; Cuevas-Mota, J.; Metzner, M.; Teshale, E.; and Garfein, R.S. Problematic use of prescription-type opioids prior to heroin use among young heroin injectors. *Subst Abuse Rehabil* 2(1):173–180, 2011.

5. Lankenau, S.E.; Teti, M.; Silva, K.; Jackson Bloom, J.; Harocopos, A.; and Treese, M. Initiation into prescription opioid misuse amongst young injection drug users.*Int J Drug Policy* 23(1):37–44, 2012.

6. Johnston, L.D.; Meich, R.A., O'Malley, P.M.; Bachman, J.G.; Schulenberg, J.E.; and Patrick, M.E. *Monitoring the Future National Results on Adolescent Drug Use: 1975-2017. Overview, Key Findings on Adolescent Drug Use.* Ann Arbor: Institute for Social Research, The University of Michigan. Available at: www.monitoringthefuture.org

7. American Psychiatric Association. *Substance-Related and Addictive Disorders, in Diagnostic and Statistical Manual of Mental Disorders*, 5th Edition. Washington, DC: American Psychiatric Publishing, 540–550, 2013.

8. National Institute on Drug Abuse, Community Epidemiology Working Group. Epidemiologic Trends in Drug Abuse, in *Proceedings of the Community Epidemiology Work Group*, January 2014, Bethesda, MD: National Institute on Drug Abuse. In preparation.

9. Waldhoer, M.; Bartlett, S.E.; and Whistler, J.L. Opioid receptors. *Annu Rev*

*Biochem* 73: 953–990, 2004.

10. Johnson, S.W.; and North, R.A. Opioids excite dopamine neurons by hyperpolarization of local interneurons. *J Neurosci* 12(2):483–488, 1992.

11. Goldstein, A. Heroin addiction: neurobiology, pharmacology, and policy. *J Psychoactive Drugs* 23(2):123–133, 1991.

12. National Library of Medicine. *Cerebral hypoxia*. Available at: https://medlineplus.gov/ency/article/001435.htm. Updated: August 29, 2012. Last accessed: October 30, 2014.

13. Wang, X.; Li, B.; Zhou, X.; Liao, Y.; Tang, J.; Liu, T.; Hu, D.; and Hao, W. Changes in brain gray matter in abstinent heroin addicts. *Drug Alcohol Depend* 126(3):304–308, 2012.

14. Ignar, D.M.; and Kuhn, C.M. Effects of specific mu and kappa opiate tolerance and abstinence on hypothalamo-pituitary-adrenal axis secretion in the rat. *J Pharmacol Exp Ther* 255(3):1287–1295, 1990.

15. Kreek, M.J.; Ragunath, J.; Plevy, S.; Hamer, D.; Schneider, B.; and Hartman, N. ACTH, cortisol and beta-endorphin response to metyrapone testing during chronic methadone maintenance treatment in humans. *Neuropeptides* 5(1-3):277–278, 1984.

16. Li, W.; Li, Q.; Zhu, J.; Qin, Y.; Zheng, Y.; Chang, H.; Zhang, D.; Wang, H.; Wang, L.; Wang, Y.; Wang, W. White matter impairment in chronic heroin dependence: a quantitative DTI study. *Brain Res* 1531:58-64, 2013.

17. Qiu, Y.; Jiang, G.; Su, H.; Lv, X.; Zhang, X.; Tian, J.; Zhou, F. Progressive white matter microstructure damage in male chronic heroin dependent individuals: a DTI and TBSS study. *PLoS One* 8(5):e63212, 2013.

18. Liu, J.; Qin, W.; Yuan, K.; Li, J.; Wang, W.; Li, Q.; Wang, Y.; Sun, J.; von Deneen, K.M.; Liu, Y.; Tian, J. Interaction between dysfunctional connectivity at rest and heroin cues-induced brain responses in male abstinent heroin-dependent individuals. *PLoS One* 6(10):e23098, 2011.

19. Kreek, M.J.; Levran, O.; Reed, B.; Schlussman, S.D.; Zhou, Y.; and Butelman, E.R. Opiate addiction and cocaine addiction: underlying molecular neurobiology and genetics. *J Clin Invest* 122(10):3387–3393, 2012.

20. Chen, L.H.; Hedegaard, H.; and Warner, M. QuickStats: Number of Deaths from Poisoning, Drug Poisoning, and Drug Poisoning Involving Opioid Analgesics - United States, 1999–2010. *Morbidity and Mortality Weekly Report* 234, 2013.

21. Magiorkinis, G.; Sypsa, V.; Magiorkinis, E.; Paraskevis, D.; Katsoulidou, A.; Belshaw, R.; Fraser, C.; Pybus, O.G.; and Hatzakis, A. Integrating phylodynamics and epidemiology to estimate transmission diversity in viral epidemics. *PLoS Comput Biol* 9(1):e1002876, 2013.

22. Centers for Disease Control and Prevention. *Viral Hepatitis Surveillance - United States*, 2010. Atlanta, GA: Centers for Disease Control and Prevention, 2012.

23. Nelson, P.K.; Mathers, B.M.; Cowie, B.; Hagan, H.; Des Jarlais, D.; Horyniak, D.; and Degenhardt, L. Global epidemiology of hepatitis B and hepatitis C in people who inject drugs: results of systematic reviews. *Lancet* 378(9791):571–583, 2011.

24. Jones, H.E.; Kaltenbach, K.; Heil, S.H.; Stine, S.M.; Coyle, M.G.; Arria, A.M.; O'Grady, K.E.; Selby, P.; Martin, P.R.; and Fischer, G. Neonatal abstinence syndrome after methadone or buprenorphine exposure. *N Engl J Med* 363(24):2320–2331, 2010.

25. Kraft, W.K.; Dysart, K.; Greenspan, J.S.; Gibson, E.; Kaltenbach, K.; and Ehrlich, M.E. Revised dose schema of sublingual buprenorphine in the treatment of the neonatal opioid abstinence syndrome. *Addiction* 106(3):574–580, 2010.

26. Lund, I.O.; Fischer, G.; Welle-Strand, G.K.; O'Grady, K.E.; Debelak, K.; Morrone, W.R.; Jones, H.E. A comparison of buprenorphine + naloxone to buprenorphine and methadone in the treatment of opioid dependence during pregnancy: maternal and neonatal outcomes. *Subst Abuse* 7:61–74, 2013.

27. Boyer, E.W. Management of opioid analgesic overdose. *N Engl J Med* 367(2):146–155, 2012.

28. Coffin, P.O.; and Sullivan, S.D. Cost-effectiveness of distributing naloxone to heroin users for lay overdose reversal. *Ann Intern Med* 158(1):1–9, 2013.

29. U.S. Food and Drug Administration. FDA approves new hand-held auto-

injector to reverse opioid overdose. *FDA News Release.* April 3, 2014. Available at http://www.fda.gov/NewsEvents/Newsroom/PressAnnouncements/ucm391465.htm.

www.ingramcontent.com/pod-product-compliance
Lightning Source LLC
Chambersburg PA
CBHW082123220526
45472CB00009B/2284